How to Be Fit and Healthy
Taking the Road Less Traveled

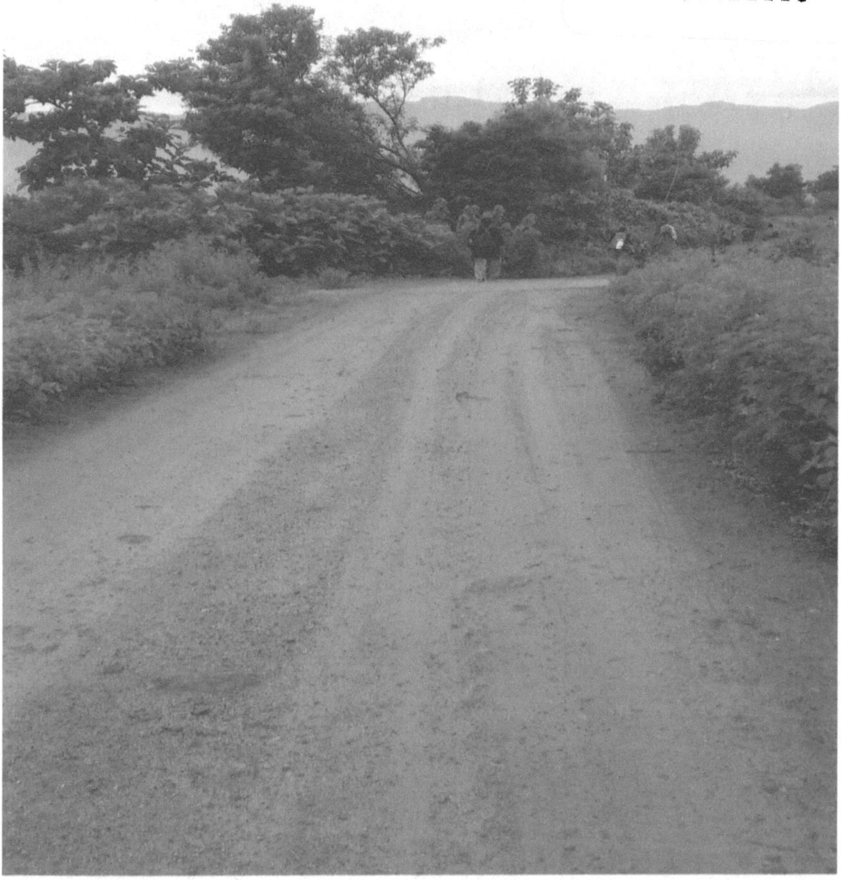

By: Charvi Nangia and Robert Cunningham

First Printing: October 12, 2017

Introduction

If you're reading this book, then you are most likely curious about one very important thing. YOUR HEALTH! It's the most important topic of all of life today. It's likely that you've discovered that a few extra pounds have caused you to feel out of sorts. Possibly those favorite jeans you found in the back of your wardrobe no longer fit like they used to? Well, for whatever reason you've come, thank goodness you found this book. Now, we're not going to sit here and deluge you with guilt about how it occurred, either through low metabolism, childbirth, over-indulgence after many years, whatever it is, we aren't here to debate or deride you, but to inform and enlighten. (If you'll pardon the pun)

The reason you bought this book was to aide you in becoming healthier and more productive in your life, am I correct? Then let's get to it, shall we?

What you hold in your hands now is not conclusive, but a simple guide to better health, energy, exercise recommendations and more. Hundreds of books have been written by others about the newest fad diets, or exercise regimens that help some, but the only real thing that gets thinner is your wallet, correct? Welcome to the world of FITNESS TRAINING and its many incarnations. Let's examine this for just a moment.

Meaning of Being Healthy

Your health is the most precious of jewels. A fit and healthy individual is the most opulent person in the world. In other words, eating a proper diet, regular workouts and taking proper care of your body is the whole essence of being healthy. This is the time when money matters are extremely important for everyone leading a luxurious lifestyle. People the world over travel around that same world seeking the best sources to earn a living, and in all of this, their health remains hidden and a mystery. Nobody even thinks of, what will you do with all the wealth of the world if you do not possess good health? What's the use of having wealth, if a maximum part of it is going to medical shops for your medicines? So, it's better to be fit than to be a regular customer of a doctor.

Good health can be attained by bringing good habits into your daily routine. With hard work and a bit of luck, being a healthy and fit individual also favors a lot in making you a successful person. Those who do, follow a different lifestyle than the rest of the crowd. To achieve great heights in your life, you need to adapt to a number of healthy practices.

Pace at Which You Should Lead Life

Getting yourself into these habits may look like a huge challenge to you. It's a tough task until you finally accustom yourself to a discipline of following healthy conducts. It is actually easy once you get into the flow. Train your mind first and your body will follow. Many of us follow the custom of making New Year's resolution promises to ourselves in the month of January like watching our diets and eating healthy all through the year; following a specific schedule including exercises, talking less on the phone and focusing more on the outside world etc. But, what happens by the end of the year?

Sometimes we don't even make it to the end of the month of January! We all know the answer to it. These resolutions are practiced only for few months. With more involvement in other things, we forget what we had promised to ourselves in the beginning of the year. We are left with remorse. There is no need to revamp your everyday life. Just try to bring in little variations, slowly. These simple changes can bring out bigger outcomes.

Being healthy means being energetic, beautiful and graceful, being noticed by everyone and living a longer life. Being in shape is not always easy but taking various directives will lead you to a healthier life. You will definitely see improvements in yourself in a short time.

Remember, being positive always helps a person in achieving anything in life and you need to think that it's not at all that tough. You can plan, and follow up on a schedule, and activities on a regular basis.

Determination and integrity serve well to see things achieved, and this is where they come into play. Setting short term goals that you can achieve, then working harder to achieve greater long term goals. Start out small, like cutting back or even replacing soft drinks with teas or juices. Cutting out salty snacks and sweets, or reducing some of the heavier foods we consume. ONE piece of cake isn't a bad thing. Eating the WHOLE cake is!

Start walking to nearby venues like the store or strolling along a pathway for a mile or so. Take up biking, or an easier sport like golf, or go dancing. Once to twice a week and these events help to maintain your body's need for exercise.

Conception

Imagine yourself looking younger and fit. Having a positive imagination will help you a lot. We're not talking about living in a fantasy, or live in an imaginary world, but with a positive visualization you can live a disease free, energetic and enthusiastic life. For this, you need to be calm, collective, and create a positive mindset. You need to take time out for yourself, sit quietly and ruminate over your goals of being healthy. Contemplate the possibilities for success. For achieving this, you need to work on various steps like eating healthier food, getting proper nutrition, doing regular exercise, working your mind as well as your muscles, etc.

Wake Up Early

We all know the famous saying- "Early to bed and early to rise makes a man healthy, wealthy and wise". -- Ben Franklin. It's very true in all of its terms, but in today's corporate world, people work in the morning, all day, and night shifts. This means they have to work at night and sleep in the morning or during the daylight hours, which is a totally different schedule. Being a night riser is not that bad if you are okay with it and its routine, but being an early riser is excellent as it has many benefits. Some of them are:

Warm Welcome of the Day

It's a new day and you need to get up and receive the day with an open heart, feeling lucky that you are alive and living a wonderful and precious life. Promise yourself that you are not going to discard this blessing of life with pettiness and sorrow, that your will for the day is one of co-operation, compassion and love for your fellow man. Feel positive about yourself and tell yourself that you will greet everyone with a warm heart.

You will be kind to others, you will not let negativity surround you, and you will work for the benefit of others. You will not get angry at anyone or say anything cruel which can hurt the other person. Feel energetic and start your day using your full potential. This is the true path to health.
Recognizing this will make the world more bearable and your days brighter and worthwhile. It is a proven fact that those who rise and greet the day with enthusiasm and warmth find it easier to deal with

stressful situations and distressing news should it come. Ask anyone who does this and they will tell you, those moments, where they just sit and take in the sunrise, are the most peaceful of their entire day. A few moments alone allows them to focus and begin the day in a right frame of mind. Don't believe me? Try it for yourself. Give it a few mornings and see what benefits you derive from it.

No Hurry

There are times when you just wake up, hopping out of the bed or maybe even the couch and are in a hurry to get ready for work and get your children ready for school. In this rush, you and your kids can be late for school and work and you might miss the amazing sunrise. You'll enter into work with a lazy and messy look which states you have not given much thought to how it affects the perception of those around you. It doesn't give a good impression of you OR your colleagues, now does it?

Now, there is another mode to start your morning, which is quite easy. You simply need to go to bed early, get some decent rest and then you will wake up on time. All of your morning chores will get over with no worry. You will be calm and your whole day will be awesome. Try it out for yourself and see if it makes a difference in your life. I guarantee this will become your routine form this point forward.

Peace Time for Yourself

Early morning is the time when there is no traffic on the road, or any pollution, and noise. There is only fresh air and serenity. According to many, it's the best time to enjoy the beauty of nature, to sit quietly and relax your mind and heart, to give time to you and to take in fresh air. You can do whatever you want according to your interests, like reading books, taking a brisk walk, exercising, enjoying a cup of coffee with your mate, yoga or other workout regimen, etc.

Mentally Fit

Waking up early has an advantage of abridging strain. When you are stressed, you'll get a lot of negative thoughts, compounded with worries and doubts. This leads to not only a bad outlook, but continued exposure to such stresses can lead to heart, liver, brain and other bodily diseases. These are proven medical facts. When you are relaxed you will be optimistic and stress can be dealt with more easily without the need for medications and their side effects to consider. Imagine how much richer you will be when you simply get up early, allow those negative thoughts and worries to drain from your body, thus allowing your body's natural healing and restoration to occur.

See the Sunrise

According to science, people who see the sun rise daily are the most fit and healthy. They are taking advantage of the natural things around them to maintain their health. The warming rays of the sun can revive your body and Vitamin D is absorbed naturally to aide in the body's needs and replenishes it. Try to see the incredible colors of nature. If you take vitamin D, do so before 9 am as after that, the sun's rays become stronger (especially during the summer months) and they might harm your skin.

Make Your Body Fit, Exercise in the Morning

You might exercise at any time suitable to you, but a workout in the morning before breakfast is the best time. The environment is calm and fresh; most people are still sleeping or just getting home from their overnight jobs. Either way it's more peaceful and relaxing, allowing you to free yourself from stress. At other times, your schedule can get canceled due to some pressing issues of the day, but in the morning the chances are less likely that you'll be called away to do something else more important.

Efficiency

This is the perfect time for productivity. Anything creative originates quickly in your mind as you feel fresh in the morning. Ideas and thoughts flow freely and allow you to make the most of them. You can complete left-over work at this time or do anything that interests you like painting, writing, studies, cooking or baking for the day, etc. After all your work is done you can give more of your precious time to your family. It's not a difficult Job. How to manage it

Rising early is not at all a tough job and you need to think the same way. Everything becomes stable after some time. You need to do it slowly. There's no need to pressure yourself. Each day, try to wake up 5 minutes earlier than your regular time and do this progressively. Put an alarm on your cell phone and try to keep it far from your bed as you have to wake up and turn off the alarm. This effort is enough to wake you up. Also, try to sleep early, only then you will be able to wake up on time. Have an aim. Do not just wake up and roam around. In the beginning, try to do something that pleases you.

Take a hot cup of tea and feel fresh. There's a saying by Benjamin Franklin "The early morning has gold in its mouth" which is very true as it has many advantages. Become a miner of that gold and find your way to a refreshing morning and new routine that will lead to a more fit and relaxed person overall.

This page left intentionally blank for notes. . . . .

Don't Be an Insider, GO Outside

In this technical world, people are more focused towards their gadgets. Your health is very precious. Going outside, taking in fresh air is much better and healthier than sitting inside the four walls of your room or work cubicle. Exercising in gyms is good, but it will be better for you health-wise, if you exercise in your local park or anywhere outside in fresh air. Running in open air will have more benefits than running in a gym.

If you woke up early, then don't think of sleeping again or don't get stuck to your gadget. Just wash off your face and get ready to meditate, run or walk. Whenever you wake up early, try doing this. Believe me; if you will follow your walking or running schedule in the morning, without all the distractions of the day creeping into it, you are going to enjoy it. Instead of the air-conditioned gym environment, try preferring an open area with fresh air. It will work wonders for you, I promise. Garden-fresh air boosts up oxygen level in your body, especially in your brain. This increases your body's abilities to function properly and allows anything that might affect you to be dealt with by the body's own natural defenses. Anti-oxidants and more vitamins allow the body to restore a great deal of damaged parts and therefore keep you healthier.

Some people prefer to go for a brisk walk daily either after or before dinner. This too, can be of great benefit to you as it allows your digestion to begin if after a meal and the body will recognize its functions better for doing this.

According to scientific research, people who expose themselves to natural surroundings are calmer as it seems to have a positive effect on their mental health. They stay happier, more focused, calm and more optimistic than other people. The color green acts as a stress buster and is refreshing and soothing for the eyes. An environment with greenery all around will help in lowering the stress level as it reduces the release of stress hormones in the body. People who are working outdoors and exercising in greener, more natural environments are fitter and happier than those who do this in an artificial setup.

I know the question that will arise in your mind- most of us live in high-tech cities; where do we find greenery and fresh air without pollution? No problem. Every large metropolitan city maintains green park zones for children and adults. They keep a separate zone for walking and other activities. So, go out and roam around your parks. Many find that pets being walked allows them not only more exercise, but socially acceptable interactions with others doing the same with their pets as well. Many a long term relationship has been brought about by this activity and even some marriages as they find common grounds through their love of animals. Speaking of animals, we should mention here that these pets provide a great deal of healthy benefits if you can manage them.

Obesity is one of the most common problems which can be easily detected but cannot be easily cured. Our routines are changing. There are no fixed times to eat food as it used to be and no time to exercise which leads to laziness and stress. Stress can boost obesity which leads to many health complications. So many things have become sedentary in their design now. Golf was designed to give you not only a competitive game but exercise as well. NOW we have motorized golf carts because we don't want to walk all over the custom designed course. I find it amazing the lengths we go to, to get away from exercise and yet, there's a multi-billion dollar exercise industry that keeps re-inventing things to mimic everyday activities like climbing stairs, lifting weights and walking.

You need to get involved in various physical activities. One of the best ways is to play some sport. Listed below are the benefits and of outdoor sports you can opt for, for your better health.

Prefer Outdoor Sports

Sports can play a crucial role in maintaining the health of a person. People who actively participate in sports are found to be more healthy and vigilant compared to people who do not play any sport. Sports act as a pre-emptive measure and stress buster as it improves both mental and physical health. It also tends to establish a routine and some form of discipline thus allowing you to maintain your fitness once established. Now I will state here and before you that I am NOT telling you to go out there and try to become a professional at any sport.

We both know that if you have some tendency towards a particular sport, it's usually discovered when you are young and able to take full advantage of the sport's unique benefits to the body. I would never conceive of someone in their 50's trying to compete with someone over half their age in any type of sport.

That would be very foolish indeed. So realize why you're adopting this sport to begin with, for the exercise and overall fitness of your own body, not to be the next sports hero to the world. Fantasies are nice, but reality can keep you from injuring yourself trying to do more than your body is able to do. THAT is the mistake so many make when they try to do sports after a lifetime of inactivity. Thinking they are able to keep up with younger people and compete.

Schools are meant to educate children, but why do they prefer to have a sports hour? Why children are taught different extra-curricular activities is beyond me. An education does not come only from books. It is meant for the overall development of a child which can be accomplished by performing various extracurricular activities, especially sports. Communal activities encourage camaraderie and discipline. Continuous studying for long hours exhausts your mind. To make it feel fresh and active you need to give it a break. So, if you have an interest in sports, go outside, and be active.

Being athletic makes you healthy and can be attractive too. Just don't fall into the trap of being a sports hero and looking for everyone else to recognize you for it. Participating in sports is made for keeping the body fit, NOT to become a wealthy, self important snob, as many who become professional sports players are today.

Find a sport that interest you and go outside! It has many perks, some are as follows:

Sound Sleep

When you play high intensity sports, it saps your body's energy and you feel tired. This is a good thing. When your body discharges energy, it requires some rest to re-energize it for the next day. A good night's sleep is very important for a body and a tired person will more likely get sound sleep. You will be more productive and creative if you sleep well.

Never try to work or operate machinery if you are too tired as this leads to many accidents and possibly death. Taking care of yourself is the key here and it should be obvious by now that we are looking to help you in that area.

This page left intentionally blank for notes. . . . .

Sunshine - Good for Your Bones

This is the corporate world and many of us have desk jobs, sit in air-conditioned offices and can't take time out for ourselves. According to the latest research, approximately one billion people of our population all over the world, including all age groups, are suffering from a deficiency of vitamin D. People do not know the benefits of exposing their body to sunlight and fresh air. Consumption of vitamin D is very important for our bones as it has lots of calcium which is essential for our whole body and it is possible only when we allow ourselves to come out of the rooms and let our body breathe in fresh air and sunlight. We've come to know of many bone problems not only in children but also in adults. Ingestion of vitamin D has many advantages and it's one of the key elements in our body. It helps the body evade lethargy, bodily disorders, and melancholy. This sunshine vitamin plays a significant role in maintaining our overall health. Some of the advantages this vitamin has are as follows below:

Scientists have proven that it has a great effect on depression which means it helps in reducing any kind of stress. Our elders keep saying this "Don't sit in darkness, sit in a bright place, and paint your room bright and not dark!" Why do they say this? The reason being darkness can lead you towards dejection. Sunshine releases antidepressants in a natural form in our brain which reduces stress level.

It can prove to be a good source of losing weight. Research shows that a body that regularly exercises gets sunshine and fresh air is less likely to be overweight as the metabolism rate is higher for those who are active and fit rather than your average couch potato. This person sees it as a regular routine, rather than a burden and inconvenience upon their day and time.

Decreases Heart Risk

When one is more active, the chances of getting heart disease are greatly lessened as the regular exercise of the muscles, of which the heart is a BIG one, keeps it functioning properly and allows you to be one step ahead of the game when it comes to being healthy. Any doctor will tell you this is true.

Congratulations, I just saved you hundreds of dollars for a doctor's visit, possible prescriptions and many years of heartaches with medical bills and hospitals. And it didn't cost you anywhere near a simple doctor's office visit or hospital stay now did it? You're welcome!

It's good in treating Alzheimer's patients. These patients become very restless especially during the night and they take a lot of stress. Research shows that exposing them to sunlight makes them less depressed and twitchy.

The brain works faster if you are exposed to sunlight daily. It is very effective for the pineal gland of the brain. An antioxidant is released by this gland which is very good for our sleep and leads to appropriate functioning of our brain.

People think that the sunshine may cause skin cancer and it is actually true. But it can only happen when you are directly exposed to mid-day sunlight. Rays of the sun are nearly harmless and soft before 12 PM, few people get sunburned early in the day.

It mostly occurs during the hours of 11 AM to 6 PM, when the concentration of the sun's rays are the highest. Careful and planned exposure can see you well protected and yet getting the nutrients and energy you need from the sun.

There is a disorder which is caused by a lesser intake of sunlight. As the seasons change, the level of depression increases. Exposure to sunlight is directly proportional to a higher level of serotonin which helps in curing this disorder named Seasonal Affective Disorder or SAD. If you are into puns it's this, "A day without sunshine makes you SAD!" Sorry, I couldn't resist that one and laughter also is good for the body, as it releases endorphins into the bloodstream that are beneficial to it. See? I not only saved you hundreds of dollars, but gave you a spiritual lesson as well. THIS is the opposite of SAD. (The Bible: King James version-Proverbs 17:22 – A merry heart doeth good like a medicine: but a broken spirit drieth the bones.)

It endorses the health of our eyes. We don't go out in sunlight because it can have a bad effect on our eyes. But let me inform you that the sunshine is not an enemy to our eyes. The sun's rays are beneficial for your vision and can also act as healing agent for many eye diseases.

Doctors say that it entices invulnerable cells towards the surface of our skin and helps in fighting many skin diseases like liver spots or bad skin (acne), eczema, psoriasis, skin cancer, scabies etc. Melatonin in our skin needs Vitamin D to maintain itself and the more we expose our bodies to the sun's healing rays, the better our health.

It should be shared here that I am neither a doctor nor a medical practitioner of any sort. The advice given herein is meant to aide you in your life, and allows YOU to make better choices for yourself with a small bit of guidance from a friend. Now that we've gotten that much cleared, let's continue shall we?

Remember that depression is a cause of many health problems one of which is weight gain. The Hypo-thalamus is a fragment of your brain that controls your hunger. The more the serotonin level in the body, the less hungry you feel. Serotonin can be multiplied by gaining sunlight daily and this can be done by your involvement in more and more outdoor activities.

It always enhances your temperament. If you are in a bad mood, then the best way to get out of it is to go outside and let your body breathe in the fresh air and sunlight. Whenever you lose your temper, try going outside and breathing deeply a few times and see the difference it makes.

Vitamin D plays a significant role in Type 2 diabetes. Diabetes is a common disease among adults. But these days it's also spreading in teenagers. Sunlight yields the body to produce a good amount of insulin in our body. Speed of production of insulin, glucose leveling, and fewer insulin conflicts are some of the positive effects of exposing a diabetes patient to sunlight.

One of the most common health problems in our world's population is High Blood Pressure. People need to take medications for their entire life to keep it controlled and normal. But, you should know that one of the best ways for treatment to the ailment of this disease is being in contact with sunlight.

The topmost layer of our skin (the dermal layer) has an element found in it called nitric oxide and when we get out in the sunlight our blood vessels become broadened and it allows for a good flow of nitric oxide in the blood which helps in lowering blood pressure. Through sweating and the removal of toxins via this layer, we keep the blood flowing at maximum efficiency thus reducing the extra strain placed upon the heart by the restricting of the veins.

Always sitting in front of the laptop or desktop and straining your eyes and mind can weaken your immune system. Solar energy increases your body's immune power and helps to strip off all kinds of toxic wastes from your body. So, it is highly advisable by experts to let your body feel the warmth of the rays of the sun for 10 – 15 minutes daily. It will definitely work in your favor. Try it for yourself and see.

There are various outdoor activities which are fun to do. Some of them are: Mountaineering, Hiking, Camping, River Rafting, Cricket, Basketball, Baseball, Skating, Swimming, Volleyball, Archery, Running, Golf, Cycling, Arts, Walking, Wrestling, Sailing, Tennis, Hockey, Sky and Water Diving, Gardening, Mind Games, Brain Teasers, Martial Arts and so many more than we could list here.

Give Less Time to Your Gadgets

Electronic gadgets like cell phones, laptops, I-Pods, I-Pads, Bluetooth, tablets, and notebooks, etc. are becoming an essential part of our growing population. We also need them, as in today's times there is very little work done manually, or by hand, everything is automatic now. Everything is on the Internet. If you want something made, order it and it will be delivered in just a few days time. Are you Hungry? Just open a can or take a meal already prepared out of the freezer, pop it into the microwave and in a few minutes you have whatever you desire.

You need to start a business; it's better to be on the Internet than to open a brick and mortar shop, assemble everything and park yourself there. You can share and promote everything on your phone via the Internet. On one hand, these gadgets are making our lives easy and more entertaining as we can do anything from the comfort of our homes.

Unfortunately activities like sitting at home, watching the news on the phone, checking Face Book, listening to songs, watching movies, doing your work, doing school studies, long distance communication with friends and family, and video calling etc. mean sitting there doing essentially NO work or physical labor. NO exercise either, means we get fat from not working those muscles and the body begins storing it up as it tries to cope with the lack of activity.

The plus point to modern conveniences is that they are handy and pocket-friendly and can be carried anywhere. It's up to YOU to determine when you have had enough of the modern appliances and start taking control of your life once more.

Here's the funny part, one of the most common phrases in the cell phone/computer/tablet world is, "There's an APP for that!" and now is no different. There are literally millions of applications out there in the world, with hundreds upon hundreds dedicated to maintaining your good health. New cell phones can monitor your heart rate, blood pressure, temperature and much more with a blue-tooth wristband tied into it.

There are Apps that allow you to keep track of your steps each day so you can judge for yourself if you're walking enough or not, it allows the device to tell the difference between walking and jogging or other activities. There are drawbacks too. Some of them are:

Obsession

I agree with the point that these devices are a great and easy source of learning especially for children but overuse of anything is not good at all. Things done within a limit are good but as they go beyond the limits, it will lead to problems. Modern day schools are using laptops instead of paper and pencil to teach children which is not a correct technique. We all know that children get attracted towards anything interesting.

They don't know how to control their attractions. Mobile phones and laptops have so many applications of games, music, drawing, photos etc. which can attract anyone. When everything is available on the phone and can be easily browsed, then why would anyone go through the trouble of going outside and looking for things they want? Game applications like superhero games, car racing, escape games, all the kind of outdoor games like cricket, football, golf, tennis, baseball, basketball, bicycling, etc. are very appealing and oftentimes one can't stop playing these games.

If you are like most people, when you start doing something interesting on the computer, you start enjoying it more and more and you will not realize that you have become a computer addict. And if you are into your gadget often enough, you will lose interest in the outer world. If you misplace or don't find your device around you, you become anxious. So, it creates a feeling of restlessness in you. Your children will lose interest in their studies and other outdoor and physical activities like sports, dance etc. and creativity will become zero. You will only want to be around your phone or laptop all the time. Connection with the outer world is very important for your health.

Isn't it ironic that the very devices we created to make our lives easier and more productive cause so many problems in our lives and make it less efficient?

Doubt that you're an addict? I have seen this MANY times on Face Book, but I believe it bears repeating.

Too many times I have seen posts wherein someone puts up a photo of a lonely middle of nowhere place with no electricity or modern facilities and asks people if they'd live there for a specified period of time, (usually 1-3 months or even a year) for a million dollars or more. Hundreds of people say YES I WOULD DO THAT!

That is until they realize that means no running water, which they will have to secure each day from a stream, river or other means. They will most likely be carrying it from the stream a few miles each way. There's no heat or Air Conditioning to keep them comfortable either and they would have to forage for their own food. Just like the settlers did in the Old West of the USA over 150 years ago. Chopping wood for fires and making sure it didn't go out or burn your house down isn't easy work. Neither is washing your clothes by hand since you won't have a washer and a dryer or laundry services to call upon. Its called MANUAL LABOR and no that's NOT hiring someone else to do it for you.

That's another thing, NO phones, NO TV or radio, NO indoor plumbing (outhouses anyone?), NO internet, NO emails, NO grocery stores, NO cars, buses or taxi's, NO neighbors to listen to or fight with, nothing but the sounds of nature all around you. IF you thought enough ahead and brought a few books, you could read them several hundred times over in that time. Would YOU fare any better? How would you face the hardships that our ancestors faced to make it in this world? Depending upon nature to feed, clothe, shelter and sustain you.

So, don't let this kind of addiction come home. Children learn faster by observing the activities of people around them and if you become a device geek then remember your children will do the same. Worst part is THEY won't know its bad for them and find a way to walk away from it.

Dependency

Electronic devices are very useful in our daily lives but it has another face too. Everything can be easily done using technology but total dependence on anything is not good for us. This technology is making us a slave to it. People are losing their power of imagination. IF your devices break down and no one has the imagination to fix them for you, then what will you do? It seems nobody wants to do anything manually anymore as the computer does it all for you. NO manual work means risking your health as the lack of physical exercise, as we've shown earlier is very detrimental to your health.

Harmful Waves

Most of these devices are electronic and wireless. This leads to exposure of harmful and invisible rays. These waves can harm any part of your body, you're your brain, your eyes, your ears etc. and can also cause deadly diseases like cancer, Alzhelmer's etc. If you keep looking into the laptop for long hours then it can have a bad effect on your eyes and can make your vision weak. Spending a lot of time listening to songs on headphones can diminish your hearing capacity and it can also make you deaf. Keeping your phone or modem 'on' the whole night can be the cause of many diseases as dangerous radiations are released during the night. So, it's better to use your devices only when needed. There is more than enough evidence available to you to prove this statement, if you need to verify it. Research is a more productive use of your time on the computer than games or shopping for items you have no need for. Just do so when you're awake and able to focus, not in the middle of the night when you can't sleep due to worries and doubt. There are studies that also show that using the phone at night when you should be sleeping interrupts the sleep pattern and you become like a zombie the next day and not working at your very best.

This page left intentionally blank for notes. . . . .

Communication Problem

Good communication skills play a very crucial role in the development of your career. Being in touch with everyone around you keeps you happy and healthy. But if you always keep digging out your phone to play on it, then you will not get the time to go outside and explore things, to communicate with people and to make new friends. Many social applications allow you to meet new people, but only online.

Your typing and chatting skills can get stronger, but face to face communication will only get weaker. You cannot know a person and call him/her your friend only by chatting on the Internet. You'll be more into texting than into communication. Communications skills rely on a face to face meeting, so that you can interpret the other person's meanings from their words and the expressions on their face. Text only can make you more introverted and soon, you will not find the need to communicate to people outside. And people who are more inclined towards themselves are found to be weaker in health compared to social people. This is why they have even come up with icons to show emotions called EMOJI's so that there is some form of emotion shown and you can better interpret the meaning of the text you are being sent.

There have been many Internet frauds in the recent years that prey upon people's naivete. It is so easy to fake paperwork, logos and even real looking documents, but a face to face meeting allows you to

SEE what the person is saying and doing while they are doing it. If technology teaches you anything, it's that good things are there for you to explore. Just like outside, there are many wonderful things to find on the internet, but you have to limit yourself to how long you expose yourself to it to allow yourself time for the really important things in your life. YOUR HEALTH! The Internet also has many bad and censored videos which can spoil your child's mind and morals. So parents, it is good for you to keep your phone locked and away from your child. This will encourage them to seek out healthy and fun activities other than sitting in their rooms simply playing games and not growing to their full potentials.

Physical Loss

According to expert doctors, if you spend long hours on your devices, it can lead to lifelong impairment in your body and its functions. This is true especially for children. Assorted computer devices like Cell Phones, I-Pads, I-Pods. Tablets and the like impair the proper development of their brain. Paper and pencil work also make their muscles stronger. Learning is an activity that strengthens their bodies and their minds. Remember, the brain is the largest muscle in the human body that has NO underlying muscles that surround it to support it. It is encased in bone, but the lack of physical activity will cause it not to develop properly and that causes more adult diseases down the road of life.

Nowadays most of the devices are touch sensitive. Excessive use of your thumb and fingers can weaken your hand muscles. It can make your hand feel numb sometimes. It is no secret that all this increases obesity as well as when one is zoned out, proper nutrition and exercise is often waived for the excitement of a game. True, it may stimulate the brain, but it only mimics the activities of the body and doesn't allow for the actual body to get any benefits.

Negative Effect on Environment

Most electronic devices are not exactly environmentally friendly. After being damaged, they are transported to far away countries like China or India. These damaged units are melted down to convert them into metals again to make more devices. This will definitely pollute the Earth. Not only the ground environment but also water resources as they often release high amounts of toxic gases.

These gases are very harmful and can lead to many respiratory diseases like asthma, influenza, Bronchitis, lung disease etc. and lead to many early deaths for those working in the factories.

Neck Pain

Sitting in a particular position for extended periods of time can cause neck and back pain as your spinal disc will be under irregular pressure. This should not be ignored. It can affect your muscles, nerves, and joints which can become a health issue later and can be a long-term problem. Your body can become easily out of shape.

Continually using your thumb and fingers to press or click on the screen can have a bad effect on your wrist and it can cause a regular pain and a malady called RSS (Repetitive Stress Syndrome). Doing everything simultaneously like watching television, working on the laptop and attending phone calls can lead to an irritated mood with not being able to concentrate on things and focus your attention as you should on tasks at hand and it will definitely affect your brain.

In earlier days, we used to write down phone numbers and remember them because our memories used to be sharp. But now, we can just save the contact in our cell phones. This also weakens our ability to think and store things in our brains as we delegate those tasks to a computer. This is demonstrated by the way we react whenever our phones malfunction and lose our data. ALL those numbers you can't get access to any longer because you don't know how to recall things from memory. This is yet another problem with technology of today that has cause problems health wise.

After research, it has been proven that people who use their phones or laptops for a few hours before going to bed will not enjoy sound sleep and it leads to restlessness the whole night. They feel lazy and less attentive in their work with a feeling of overall disconnectedness. A Good and calm night's sleep always improves your health. It has been shown that people who don't spend as much time on their devices are more active. Sleeplessness can have many negative consequences like diabetes, weight gain, heart disease, stress management issues, high blood pressure, liver problems, etc.

So, the best thing you can do for yourself is to keep your phone away from you and your child and use it only when required. Remember to sit in a correct posture when working on the laptop. Don't lean too much, sit straight and relax your eyes. Take a nap of at least 15 minutes or don't focus on an object for more than a few minutes.

Travel

Traveling is the best part of life. It lets you know different places, people, and cultures. You go outside from the same environment to a totally different surrounding. There are many advantages of being a traveler. Some of them are:

Increases Contentment

Your happiness increases just by planning for a trip. Preparing to meet new people and open yourself up to new cultures, foods and places. You get the self-satisfaction of having achieved something. It's not easy to go to a totally new place among new people. Anything can also happen to you, but good planning ensures you are prepared to meet these challenges head-on. And you return safely knowing a lot more about that place, its people and its customs.

Increased Immunity

Our immune system gets stronger if we are exposed to some dust and dirt of a foreign land. The more you explore to keep yourself protected, the more your body will get prone to resist diseases. Your immune system is protected from pathogens by antibodies. This doesn't mean that you shouldn't pay attention towards hygiene. Your body should get accustomed to external bacteria so that it can effectively deal with it and not make you sick.

Positive Effect on Brain Health

Being busy with your work all the time makes your life monotonous and your mind dull. Going to a new place and discovering new things will lead to a creative mind. Traveling opens you up and makes you experience a lot of new things. Every place has its own climate and culture. You get to know new people and how they adapt to their culture. You come to like and understand people emotionally too and it makes you more global, emotionally stable and you understand another country's heritage. Science has proved that traveling increases your personal growth, inspiration, and resourcefulness. It also allows you the freedom to expand your mind with the new information and ideas that can come from a trip to foreign lands.

Fitness

Traveling can make you exhausted but also it can make you fit. You get a lot of opportunities to discover yourself. If you travel only for comfort in luxury hotels then it's a total waste. You need to get out and explore every part of a place and experiment new activities. Walking into the city will make your muscles tight and strong and spending time on a beach will make you feel relaxed. Your body will work faster. This frequenting of exercise will allow the body yo maintain itself in ever aspect of life and health

Long Life

As is proven by scientific research, travel improves your brain, lowers depression level and keep you fit physically and mentally. All this leads to a longer life. The more you travel, the more you enjoy living.

Places Which Will Improve Your Health

Nature is full of surprises and it keeps awing you every time you go to a new location. Natural springs in places like Rishikesh in India, Lourdes in France, The Wailing Wall in Jerusalem, Israel, Stonehenge in England, Steam Spa's in Iceland, Mineral Springs all over the U.S. and Turkey have lots of curative properties and can be a good medication to any of your skin diseases. There are numerous hot springs at different places which heal any type of pain in your body- whether it's a joint pain, neck or back pain. They also make you feel relaxed after a long travel. Some places are blessed with natural energy points like Mount Desert Island, Stonehenge in England, (as mentioned before) The Pyramids of Ghazi in Egypt, the best known Latin American pyramids include The Pyramid of the Sun and the Pyramid of the Moon at Teotihuacan in central Mexico, the Castillo at Chichen Itza in the Yucatan Peninsula, the Great Pyramid in the Aztec capitol of Tenochtitlan, the Great Pyramid at Cholula, and the Inca's great temple at Cuzco in Peru as well. It helps you rejuvenate your energy. All of these places are covering the world that is yours to discover and find the wonderful powers that they possess.

Lowers Heart Risk

Traveling is the best stress booster. If you are not well and taking rest for the entire day inside the four walls of a room, you will feel more weak and ill. You will want to get outside whether doctors allow it or not. And believe me, by getting outside of that room and looking at the green environment around you will help boost your health and you will recover soon. The reason is going outside and seeing new locations lowers your stress level.

Healthy Eating Habits

This is the most important step towards staying healthy and fit. It's not an easy task but not that hard either. You simply need to be determined and controlled. There is a saying by a very famous London based English writer on eating healthy. "One cannot think well, love well, and sleep well if one has not dined well". -- Virginia Woolf.

Most of us think that eating healthy means constantly dieting or you need to go on a diet to be slim and in shape. This is a big myth and you need to get out of that type of thinking. Dieting all the time will never work as you find yourself cheating from guilt and will always lead to negative results. A diet implies many constraints on you and limits your food. First of all, you need to understand that being healthy does not mean losing weight. It includes your overall health physically and mentally.

Overall health includes your inner and outer body and it needs to be fit. For this, you need to develop a new living style and eating habits. Find out what keeps you from being healthy and decide to change those habits to better yourself, without any drastic pills or vitamins that never seem to work. Worse yet, having surgery to remove the weight quickly and finding it puts your health at risk even further as it is a quick fix, but isn't always the right choice for you. Many are the people who wish they had chosen a slower means of finding the right answer instead of surgery.

Laparoscopic (Or LAP BAND surgery as it's known) sounds like a quick fix but the side effects are the months wherein you cannot eat more than a few spoonfuls of baby food for each meal until you get accustomed to lowered intake as they reduce the size of your stomach, and subsequent surgery will remove that excess portion altogether. All told it's a two year process that many wish they'd never had done as it is very shocking the changes in your life this surgery will require. Going out to eat during this time is nearly impossible as they won't have anything that's pureed on the menu that you would enjoy. Would you pay $15 for a steak that you had to put into a blender turn into a meat shake and could only eat a few spoonfuls of before you weren't able to eat anymore?

Fitness Diet

You should know your body and should be aware of food that suits you and those that you are allergic to. Eating the right kind of food is very crucial for your health. Your skin, body organs, and everything is related to good food.

It's not that occasional candy bar that throws everything out of whack with your body, as those sugars are quickly absorbed and put into use as quickly as possible for the energy is converted purely from the sugar. Fat on the other hand is stored and takes more to convert to energy than sugars as it is more complex having been converted to begin with by the body.

Getting the body to ramp up the inner fires if you will or the metabolism as it is called is what is needed to lose weight. Convincing the body that those fat cells are needed to burn for fuel to keep the body working properly is what a diet is supposed to do for you. What it really does is convince the body that those times are lean and that every effort to reserve those stored cells should be made. This is why so many diets fail. The body is at war with itself. The mind says to use the reserves and the body says. "NO we need that in case of famine or disaster! WE have to survive on that for an undetermined amount of time."

Cook For Yourself

Everybody knows that home cooked food tastes better. I agree with the fact that after working long hours, you get tired and you want someone to cook for you. This is why people hire cooks or go to restaurants or fast food places. But you should also be aware that maids and cooks are working at your house because they want to earn a living too. They will not try to cook healthy and delicious food for you every day unless instructed and paid well to do so and cooking food should not be a job.

Many of the housemaids one would hire don't care about hygiene. They clean as quickly and do as small amount of work as possible.

Even if you were to hire a professional chef for your daily meals, they look at it as a job and will do only what is asked of them, so it will still be better for you and your family to eat the meals prepared by someone from the family. If you cook for yourself, you will do it from your heart and apply every effort to prepare a delicious and healthy meal for your family members. Hygiene will be your priority as unhygienic food can lead to many infections. This would lead to doctors' visits or sickness that means going to a hospital or even worse. You'll keep in mind the exact amount of every nutrient which is good for your body and what foods will give you and your family these things daily. It will help you maintain your weight. Cooking food for your own family will always make you feel good. As you have to do it every day, you can make it interesting instead of being monotonous.

You can ask each member of your family their choice of food and prepare a single meal among many choices and keep other favorite selections for other days of the week. This way you can prepare different dishes every day. Keep things organized. Plan ahead and cooking will not be such an issue for you.

Daily Breakfast

Do you know why we call the morning meal a breakfast? Because our body takes rest the whole night digesting the meals and in the morning we break the fast by eating something that can calm down our hunger. That's why we call it breakfast. It is a kind of a fuel that your body needs to be active the whole day. One of the most popular nutritionists and author of American origin wrote a perfect quote about three meals of the day.

"Eat breakfast like a king, lunch like a prince, and dinner like a pauper." – Adelle Davis

So, fill up your body with a hearty and heavy meal at breakfast as your lunch will be a little lighter and dinner will be the least heavy meal of the day.

Eat Early and On Time

Breakfast should be done before 8:00 am as your stomach can digest it by lunch time. The notion of skipping breakfast is not a good one. People think that breakfast can be skipped. This will lead to excessive cravings. Finally you will end up eating more than what you should. Scientific research has proven that early breakfast prevents diseases and problems like obesity.   The perfect time for lunch is between 1:00 pm – 2:00 pm. There should be minimum 4-5 hours difference between every meal so that the body takes its time for digestion. Lunch should contain grains, proteins, and vegetables. It should be a little lighter than breakfast.

In the evening, you can have snacks such as cookies or salted snacks or a soda, milk, tea etc. and the last meal, which is dinner, should contain either salad or grains and vegetables with a smaller portion of meats or fishes. The appropriate time for an evening meal is between 6:00 pm– 7:00 pm and should be done 4 – 5 hours before going to bed. Your bed time should be around 10:00 pm – 11:00 pm according to which the dinner timings mentioned above are perfect.

Which Foods to Include

Eating a well-balanced diet is essential for your health. You need to remove all the useless calories from your diet. Fast foods like pizza, burgers, noodles, pasta, sandwiches and the like are the most dangerous. They are only good for your tastes and not your stomach and can be one of the leading causes of weight gain. Excesses of these foods can be very detrimental to your overall health. In moderation, an occasional treat of these types of food won't upset your diet. You should cut off all the oily and fatty foods, refined sugar, effervescent drinks, synthetic colors and flavors in any kind of processed foods. MSG and other preservatives are very harmful to the body as well. The food should be preserved, not deadly with unknown chemicals. Try to eat more natural raw foods. You can include fruits, vegetables, milk, organic foods, stuffs rich in fiber and omega 3 fatty acids. Bad choices and unhealthy eating practices can lead to many diseases like hypertension, food poisoning, diabetes, obesity and much more.

On the other side, strong and healthy eating habits will increase your immunity and make you energetic. Don't forget to eat three meals a day and never skip any of these. The following things can be had on a regular basis:

Fruits

Apples- Are a great source of fiber called pectin, which has many advantages and is rich in vitamin C. It makes your teeth whiter, is a good treatment for most of the types of cancers known, decreases cholesterol levels and keeps your heart in good health, they are good for vision, help to protect from diabetes, helps in weight loss and in treating constipation, and finally enhances the immunity system.

Oranges- Of course! Couldn't compare them if we didn't include these now could we? Besides the obvious Vitamin C, they also contain many more nutrients and vitamins, like The B Complex of Vitamins, and Oranges are a good source of several vitamins and minerals, especially vitamin C, thiamin, folate and potassium.

Vitamin C: Oranges are an excellent source of vitamin C. One large orange can provide over 100% of the daily recommended intake

Thiamin: One of the B-vitamins, also called vitamin B1. Found in a wide variety of foods.

Folate: Also known as vitamin B9 or folic acid, folate has many essential functions and is found in many plant foods.

Potassium: Oranges are a good source of potassium. High intake of potassium can lower blood pressure in people with hypertension and has beneficial effects on cardiovascular health. Oranges are rich in various bio-active plant compounds. Plant compounds are believed to be responsible for many of the beneficial health effects of oranges. The two main classes of antioxidant plant compounds in oranges are carotenoids and phenolics (phenolic compounds).

Phenolics: Oranges are an excellent source of phenolic compounds, especially flavonoids, which contribute to most of their antioxidant properties.

Hesperidin: A citrus flavonoid that is one of the main antioxidants found in oranges. It is associated with several health benefits.

Anthocyanins: A class of antioxidant flavonoids found in blood oranges, which makes their flesh red. Carotenoids: All citrus fruits are rich in carotenoids, a class of antioxidants that is responsible for their orange color. Beta-cryptoxanthin: One of the most abundant carotenoid antioxidants is found in oranges. The body is able to convert it into vitamin A.

Lycopene: An antioxidant found in high amounts in red-fleshed navel oranges (Cara cara oranges). It is also found in tomatoes and grapefruit and has various health benefits.

Citric Acid: Oranges, Lemons, Limes. Grapefruits, and other fruits of the citrus family, are high in citric acid and citrates, which contribute to the sometimes sour taste. Research indicates that citric acid and citrates from oranges may help prevent kidney stone formation. Oranges are a rich source of several antioxidants that are responsible for many of their health benefits. Health Benefits of Oranges- Studies in both animals and humans indicate that regular consumption of oranges is associated with various health benefits.

Heart Health

Heart disease is currently the world's most common cause of premature death. Flavonoids in oranges, especially hesperidin, may have protective effects against heart disease. Clinical studies in humans have found that daily intake of orange juice for 4 weeks has a blood-thinning effect and may reduce blood pressure significantly. Fibers also seem to play a part. Intake of isolated fibers from citrus fruits has been shown to decrease blood cholesterol levels. Taken together, it is likely that regular consumption of oranges may help lower the risk of heart disease. As a good source of antioxidants and fiber, oranges may cut the risk of heart disease.

Prevention of Kidney Stones

Oranges are a good source of citric acid and citrates, which are believed to help prevent kidney stone formation. Potassium citrate is often prescribed to patients with kidney stones.

Citrates in oranges seem to have similar effect. Being a rich source of citric acid and citrates, oranges may help prevent kidney stone formation.

Prevention of Anemia

Anemia, the decrease in the amount of red blood cells or hemoglobin in the blood, is often caused by iron deficiency. Although oranges are not a good source of iron, they are an excellent source of organic acids, such as vitamin C (ascorbic acid) and citric acid. Both vitamin C and citric acid can increase the absorption of iron from the digestive tract. Therefore, when eaten with iron-rich food, oranges can help prevent anemia. Oranges are not rich in iron. However, when eaten with iron-rich food, they may contribute to improved iron absorption and reduce the risk of anemia.

Whole Oranges vs. Orange Juice

Orange juice is a very popular drink throughout the world. One of the main differences between orange juice and whole oranges, is that juice is much lower in fiber. This decrease in fiber seems to increase the glycemic index slightly. A cup of orange juice has a similar amount of natural sugar as two whole oranges and is much less fulfilling.

As a result, fruit juice consumption can often become excessive and may contribute to weight gain and harmful effects on metabolic health. Quality orange juice can be healthy in moderation, but whole oranges are generally a much better choice. Eating whole oranges is generally healthier than drinking orange juice.

Fruit juices tend to be high in sugar, and not as filling as whole fruit. In short, oranges don't have many known adverse effects in healthy people. Some people have an allergy to oranges, but this is rare. In people who suffer from heartburn, consumption of oranges may make symptoms worse. This is because oranges contain organic acids, mainly citric acid and ascorbic acid (vitamin C). Being among the world's most popular fruits, oranges are both tasty and nutritious. They are a good source of vitamin C, and several other vitamins, minerals, and antioxidants. For this reason, they may cut the risk of heart disease and kidney stones. Simply put, oranges are an excellent addition to a healthy eating life choice.

Avocados are a very rich source of natural fatty acids and it has various minerals and almost 20 vitamins in it like vitamin C, potassium, folate, vitamin K, vitamin B5 and B6 and vitamin E. It is good for heart, eyes, and digestion, protects against many types of cancers and serious diseases like blood pressure, heart stroke, diabetes etc., keeps your bones strong as it has lots of vitamin K, a stress booster, healthy for pregnant women as it contains folate, and they help in detoxification of the body.

Blueberries are considered a super food by many people. They are very small in size but their effects are very big. It is a highly nutritious and fibrous fruit with low calories. It contains Manganese, Vitamin C, and Vitamin K.

It protects you from aging, bone diseases, cancer, heart disease, urinary infections and damaging of muscles, decreases blood pressure, is the highest antioxidant among all foods, is a great antibiotic, sharpens your memory and maintains the appropriate level of cholesterol in the blood.

Kiwis are of the house of antioxidants and a rich source of Vitamin C, Vitamin E, B6, B12, Vitamin A, calcium, potassium, magnesium, and iron. This fibrous fruit helps in the treatment of people suffering from sleeping syndromes, fights depression and high blood pressure, good for digestion, rich in foliate, helps to boost your immunity and helps in maintaining beautiful skin.

Apricots / Peaches

These are a rich source of Vitamin A and high in fiber. They play a significant role in strengthening your bones, they are for your heart, they help purify the blood and rejuvenate your skin.

Tomatoes (YES they are a fruit) are a source of many vitamins and nutrients. Tomatoes are also an excellent source of Vitamin C, biotin, molybdenum and Vitamin K. They are also a very good source of copper, potassium, manganese, dietary fiber, Vitamin A (in the form of Beta-Carotene), Vitamin B-6, Lycopene, Folate, Niacin, Vitamin E, and Phosphorous.

VEGETABLES

These items allow for needed nutrients and anti-oxidants to be absorbed by the body, Sweet Potatoes, Carrots, Turnips, Beets, Potatoes, Radishes, Broccoli, Bracco-Flower, Cauliflower, Parsnips, and Rutabagas.

Green Leafy Vegetables

Like all forms of Lettuce, Cabbage, Broccoli, Kohlrabi, Spinach, Kale, Collard & Mustard Greens, Asparagus, Brussels' Sprouts, Bell Peppers, Broccoli Rabe.

Grains

Like Jasmine, Brown, Wild and White Rice, Barley, Wheat, Corn, Oats, Spelt, Teff, Kamut, Quinoa, and Millet.

Seafood

Items such as Salmon, Oysters, Shrimp, Whiting, Tuna, Red Snapper, Sea Bass, Flounder, Muscles, Cod, Scallops, Mackerel, Lobster, Tilapia, Eel, Octopus, Blind Robbins [from which sardines are made], Clams and Crab. (Freshwater fish include Bass, Trout, Carp, Catfish, Muskellunge, Chinook salmon, Gar Pike, and Sunfish [commonly called Bluegills] and should you like them craw fish)

Nuts

Nuts such as Almonds, Walnuts, Pistachios, Chestnuts, Cashews, Hazelnuts, Peanut, Pecan, Brazil Nuts, Pine Nuts, Water Chestnut, Filberts.

Dairy Products

Dairy Products such as Milk, Yogurt, Sour Cream, Cottage Cheese, Assorted Cheeses from around the world and eggs from many different birds, not just chickens. There are several sources of Dairy Products to choose from as well. Cows, goats, camel, sheep, oxen, even some buffalo's are milked if raised in captivity.

Bulb Vegetables

Garlic, and its close relatives including the onion, shallot, leek, chive, Bok Choy, and Chinese Onion.

Legumes include Alfalfa, Clover, Peas, Beans, (Lima, Navy, Pinto, White, Black and Cannellini), Chickpeas, Lentils, Lupin, Mung, Mesquite, Carob, Soy, Peanuts and Tamarind.

Oils

Such as olive oil, coconut oil, palm oil, soybean oil, canola oil (rapeseed oil), corn oil, peanut oil and other vegetable oils, food grade essential oils, as well as animal-based oils like butter and lard.

Keep Quantity of Processed Food Very Small

A grocery store contains a lot of items. Many fresh foods, but a great many packaged and preserved foods like bread, milk, yogurt, canned and pre-packaged meals and vegetables too. These foods go through a lot of chemical processing to which they add sugar, salt and other preservatives in the items being canned or processed. This increases the harmful effects on the body and nutrients become nil. Our body needs more nutrients to feel energetic the whole day. The preservatives used in the frozen foods and boxed meals are sometimes artificial which can be hazardous to your health. So, try avoiding boxed or frozen items and buy perishable foods which will be easy to prepare and for digestion to keep your body fueled up.

Check the Labels on Food Items

Most every edible item in the market is now available with nutrition labels to help you be aware of the nutrients in the product. They tell you the count of calories, the amount of saturated fat, salt, and sugar. It's an easy task to read these and you should always look on the label of the item before purchasing it.

Look for items with as few chemicals you can't pronounce and items that you may have allergies to like dyes and preservatives. Red #'s 3,5 & 40, Yellow's #5 & 6, Blue #'s 1 & 2 Green # 3 are the worst for allergic reactions in many people and comprise much of the coloring of boxed and packaged foods today. Fortunately today there is a concentrated effort to replace these with more natural coloring and remove as much artificial as possible from our food sources.

Always Keep Some Light Snacks

Always keep some home-made, light and healthy snacks ready. Delicious dishes like salad, pie, cookies, dried fruits, chopped and peeled carrots with a dipping sauce and pastries can be prepared using fruits, nuts, grains, and vegetables. This is for those sudden cravings when you'll be tempted to grab a package of potato chips, sugary drinks, highly caffeinated drinks, a candy bar or French fries.

Eat When Your Stomach Asks You To

Remember to never keep your stomach hungry. Whenever you feel like eating then go for a little quantity of food or drink water. Mostly, after 3-4 hours we start feeling hungry and it increases our stress level. Our body releases a hormone called cortisol when your stress level rises. And the more the cortisol level, the more fat will get deposited in your abdominal area. Don't think that skipping meals will make you slim; it always leads to high cortisol which leads to weight gain.

Eating more often in a day will stop your cravings for your favorite foods.

Eat Your Favorites Once in a While

You know that if your favorite food is on the table, you cannot stop yourself from having it and possibility is that you will have it in large quantity. This will definitely increase your weight. For a little taste, you will spoil your whole diet. So, try to eat your favorite stuff less often as it is not the last time you are going to have it.

Control Your Cravings

A fit and healthy person will never keep his/her kitchen full of chips, chocolates, ice cream, cookies, cheese, mayonnaise, cold-drinks etc. You will always see fruits, green........................ vegetables, nuts, milk etc. in their kitchen. They may have a few of these items in it, and actually know how to resist. And most importantly, you have to be determined if you seriously want to lose weight and stay healthy

Be Aware of Hazardous Foods

I mentioned above about the frozen foods which are actually dangerous if taken everyday. Foods like tomato sauces, juices etc. contain high amount of preservatives which can have a negative impact on your health. The amount of chemicals that are used to preserve and the other uses they are used for would seriously make you reconsider the foods you eat today.

Take for instance Limoline, It's a common food additive, but it's also used as a cleansing agent because it has a great amount of oils that clean dirt and other soils. So would you eat an industrial cleaner? IF you have this in any of your foods, then you are already doing so. Glycol Phosphate is another one as well. And some of the additives are one genetic sequence away from bleach! Breads use bleaching of their flours to be made white, soft, and fluffy.

Start Using Smaller Plates

It's very simple logic that you can fill up a bigger plate with a larger quantity of food at one time and you end up eating more even if not required. Whereas, a small plate will let you take on lesser amounts therefore you eat lesser calories.

Don't Over-Eat

Always try to take lesser amounts of food on your plate than what you think you need. Do not fill your plate up because it's your favorite or you are starving. There is a possibility that in the end, you are just eating to finish the food and not to calm down your hunger. This is what over-eating is which won't work towards weight loss.

Chew Properly

Do not eat like it's a race and you have to win it. Eat your food relishing its taste and in a relaxed manner.

According to research, it is found that people who eat slowly are slimmer than fast eaters as slow eating keeps your digestion good and fast eating just fills up your stomach quickly, not allowing your stomach time to process it properly.

Hydration

This is the most significant part of staying young and healthy. An adult human body contains up to 60% water. There are many fluids available in the market and also natural liquids but nothing can replace water. It is the best drink for keeping you active and healthy. It cleans our body parts and increases digestion. It also helps in washing all the toxins out of the body via urine and skin. Drinking water makes your skin feel rejuvenated. Liquids does not mean soda, cold drinks, tea, coffee, iced tea etc. Every human's body has a different capacity so, you should drink water according to your body type but drinking 8 – 10 glasses of water daily is highly recommended for everyone and will never affect your body negatively.

Exercise Commendably

Exercise is on the top of the list of staying fit. You might be having lot of other work but if you are not fit then how will you be able to complete those tasks? So, always give time to yourself for your fitness. You need to maintain a daily routine and to commit to yourself that you will definitely follow the routine in spite of being busy.

Follow the Schedule

You need to make a daily routine for your exercises. Many people join a gym for a scheduled exercise where trainers can help you. And when it comes to practice you can do it on your own at your place. Experts recommend exercising for a minimum of 30 minutes every day. So, take a few minutes out from your busy schedule and go for it.

Making It a Habit

You can select your favorite form of exercise and practice it daily. Push-ups, pull-ups, lifting weights and others are not the only exercises but any kind of physical activity which makes your body sweat and apply force like dancing, swimming, running, walking, cycling, hiking, and aerobics like ZUMBA and Pilates can be practiced.

Always wear comfortable and sweat absorbent clothes while exercising. There is a new device launched in the market named fit bit which can tell you the details of every exercise about how many calories you have burnt, how many miles or kilometers you covered while walking, your heart rate and even your sleep mode. You can opt for this gadget and can make your practice more interesting. It will even connect to your I-Phone with the application that keeps track of such things for you via a Blue Tooth connection.

Enjoy Your Exercise

You can join group exercises. This makes your training more fun. In a group, you get to know many new people. And group work is always exciting and interesting. You can listen to music according to your mood and exercise, which will maintain your tempo and will also add to fun.

Trainers always motivate you to practice every form of exercise in the best possible way you can. So, if you should have such an opportunity, be grateful that you are practicing under an expert and applying every effort to stay fit.

This page left intentionally blank for notes. . . . .

Effective Workouts

Always remember few things before doing any kind of workout. Never do any kind of exercise immediately after having a meal as it will not allow the flow of oxygen in your body. Always warm-up your body before exercising and do stretching as it will open up your body muscles and will cause less pain after a workout. Always look for a good trainer and go for an expert as any kind of wrong exercise or posture can have a negative effect on your body.

Push-ups

Lie on your stomach with your face down. You need to keep your palms on the floor and arms straight. Keep your knees straight and feet together. Move your body up and down at the arms. This should lift your upper torso. This will apply pressure on your shoulders and chest and helps you maintain a balanced body and increase the density of muscles.

Planks

Keep your hands in the similar position as in push-ups. Your body should be in a straight line. Look towards the floor and keep still. It will reduce the risk of spinal injury and improves your metabolism, posture, and flexibility.

Squat

Keep your feet a little apart. Keep your body straight. Let your knees go half down and heels should be a little off the floor. This will apply pressure on your thighs and make your leg muscles strong.

Glute Bridge

You need to lie down on your back. Your feet should be horizontal on the ground. Give a push with your heels and lift your back. This exercise will strengthen your back and leg muscles. Also, it tightens up your stomach and allows proper blood flow in the body.

Squat Jump/Thrust

Keep yourself in the same position as in a normal squat. Keep your hands straight and tight in front of you. Push it back with your jump. Your weight should be on your toes. This exercise is very effective for your thighs and stomach. A variation on this is called a Squat Thrust in which the same position is begun; only the legs are thrust to the rear in a quick fashion and you land upon your toes, legs fully extended behind you for a full three seconds then return to the starting position.

Side Lunge

Stand up straight and move your weight back and forth with your heel. Swipe your leg first on one side and then on the other. Proceed to lower yourself each time until you have gone as low as you can possibly go down without falling or injuring yourself. This exercise is good for your legs and makes them sturdier. It also improves your balance.

Yoga

Yoga is the ancient form of exercise which helps in maintaining the body, mind and soul balance. It is the easiest way to reduce your weight, curing many diseases, increasing flexibility and relieving stress. It stretches your body in several methods. Here is the list of few yoga positions:

Suryanamaskar (Salutation to the Sun)

Bhujangasana (Pose of Cobra)

Tadasana (The Mountain Posture)

Matasyasana (The Fish Pose)

Kapalabhati (Fast Inhaling and Exhaling of your breath)

Dhanurasana (The posture of a Bow)

Uttanasana (Folding down standing straight)

Baddha Konasana (Sitting in a bound position)

Trikonasana (The shape of a Triangle)

Sirsasana (Headstand)

Meditation (Lotus Position)

Eagle Twist (Wings spread out to focus energy)

What Your Body Says

Always know your body type and try to understand what it demands. "Listen to your body if you need rest. You are the best person to understand your body and what it needs." – Brennan

Never torture yourself during training. Just keep everything balanced. Be social, go outside, meet new people, make a friends circle and keep traveling. Keep yourself busy with your work, exercise, family, and friends. Believe me, you will definitely feel active and healthier. Write all your achievements and sorrows in a diary which will give you mental satisfaction and allow you to look back and judge the progress you've made in your journey to fitness. Keep your surroundings clean and always keep in mind that unhygienic conditions can lead to many diseases. Make promises to your self that you will meditate daily, avoid any carbonated drinks and bad habits of smoking and alcohol. Always think and speak positively and always eat healthy. Keep visiting your doctor for regular check-ups. Your health is your asset and you are the ONLY one who can take care of your body in the best possible way. Stay healthy, fit and HAPPY!

Charvi Nangia

&

Robert Cunningham

This book is among a series of DIY and Self help books by Khinsharri Publishing with the cooperation of Charvi Nangia, an East India native who has put a great deal of her beliefs, body and soul into this publication.

Robert Cunningham is an author, writer, ghost writer, proofreader, editor, and publisher of many styles of books and genres of fiction.

Thank you for reading this book and please look for our other books in this genre. They may be found on Amazon.com

In order to keep pricing and such to a minimum and allow as many people as possible to benefit from it, Ms. Nangia has decided NOT to include any photos or illustrations in this version of the books. Future versions MAY include these items, at the discretion of the writers/authors.

www.ingramcontent.com/pod-product-compliance
Lightning Source LLC
Chambersburg PA
CBHW012254240726
48655CB00009B/3312